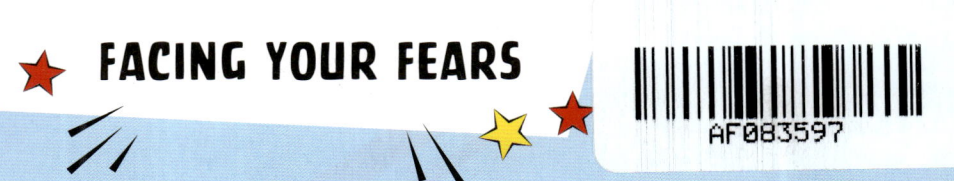

FACING YOUR FEAR OF FLYING

BY HEATHER E. SCHWARTZ

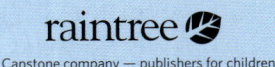

a Capstone company — publishers for children

Raintree is an imprint of Capstone Global Library Limited, a company incorporated in England and Wales having its registered office at 264 Banbury Road, Oxford, OX2 7DY – Registered company number: 6695582

www.raintree.co.uk
myorders@raintree.co.uk

Hardback edition © Capstone Global Library Limited 2023
Paperback edition © Capstone Global Library Limited 2024
The moral rights of the proprietor have been asserted.

All rights reserved. No part of this publication may be reproduced in any form or by any means (including photocopying or storing it in any medium by electronic means and whether or not transiently or incidentally to some other use of this publication) without the written permission of the copyright owner, except in accordance with the provisions of the Copyright, Designs and Patents Act 1988 or under the terms of a licence issued by the Copyright Licensing Agency, 5th Floor, Shackleton House, 4 Battle Bridge Lane, London SE1 2HX (www.cla.co.uk). Applications for the copyright owner's written permission should be addressed to the publisher.

Edited by Donald Lemke
Designed by Sarah Bennett
Original illustrations © Capstone Global Library Limited 2023
Picture research by Julie DeAdder
Production by Katy LaVigne
Originated by Capstone Global Library Ltd

978 1 3982 4877 9 (hardback)
978 1 3982 4876 2 (paperback)

British Library Cataloguing in Publication Data
A full catalogue record for this book is available from the British Library.

Acknowledgements
We would like to thank the following for permission to reproduce photographs: Getty Images: Ariel Skelley, 14, baona, 4, Digital Vision, 10, Hispanolistic, 11, 19, Images By Tang Ming Tung, 13, Keith Brofsky, 21, ViewStock, 17, yenwen, 16; Shutterstock: aappp, 7, Diana Taliun, 20 (books), Domira (background), cover and throughout, Gorodenkoff, 9, Kapitosh (cloud), cover and throughout, Marish (brave girl), cover and throughout, muratart, cover, Nadiia Korol, 20 (doll), Olena Yakobchuk, 5, 15, Tatiana Popova, 20 (toy car), Thammanoon Khamchalee, 20 (backpack)

Every effort has been made to contact copyright holders of material reproduced in this book. Any omissions will be rectified in subsequent printings if notice is given to the publisher.

All the internet addresses (URLs) given in this book were valid at the time of going to press. However, due to the dynamic nature of the internet, some addresses may have changed, or sites may have changed or ceased to exist since publication. While the author and publisher regret any inconvenience this may cause readers, no responsibility for any such changes can be accepted by either the author or the publisher.

Printed and bound in India

CONTENTS

Taking a flight 4

Reasons to relax 6

Calming your fears 12

Enjoy the ride.. 18

    Pack a carry-on bag 20

    Glossary 22

    Find out more 23

    Index 24

    About the author.......................... 24

Words in **bold** are in the glossary.

TAKING A FLIGHT

Have you ever flown on a plane? Flying is exciting. It can feel scary too. Sometimes it's hard to tell the difference. Both feelings may make your heart race. But facing your fears can help you to feel better.

Many people are afraid to fly. It's OK to be scared. You can still take steps to have a good flight.

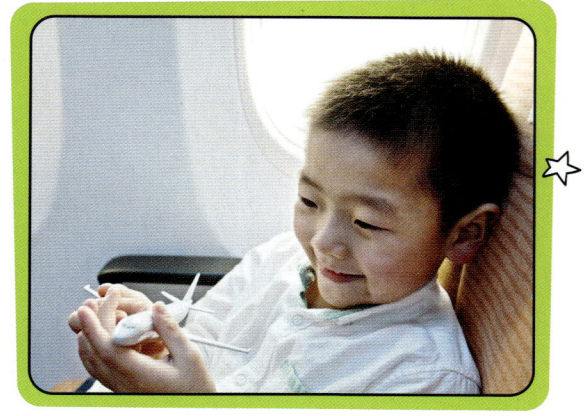

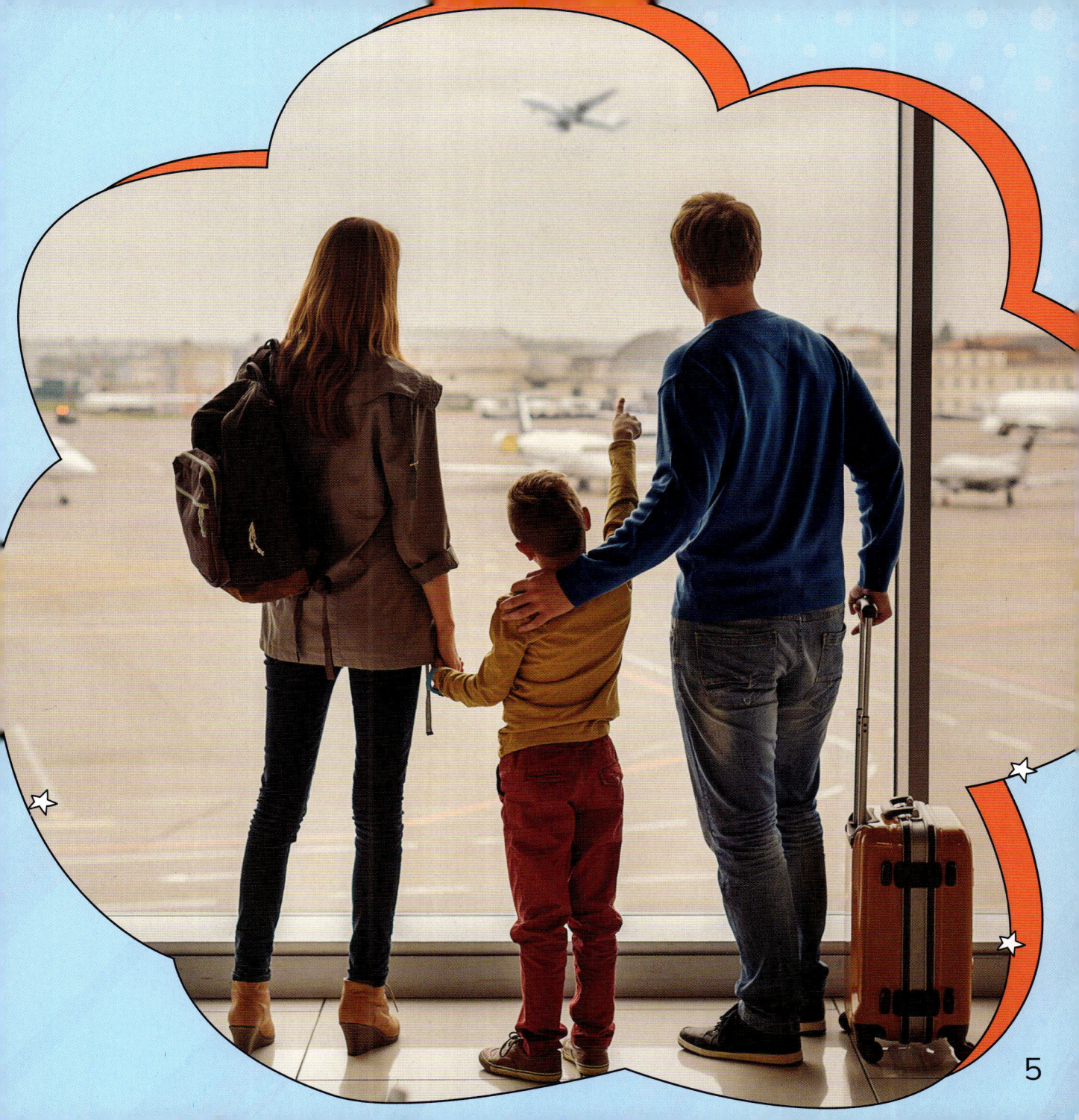

REASONS TO RELAX

Understanding how planes work can help you to relax. The engines power the plane into the sky. The air moves around the wings to keep it there.

Plane engines can be noisy. They can sound scary when they start up. But they get quieter after **take-off**. The engines will get louder again when you land.

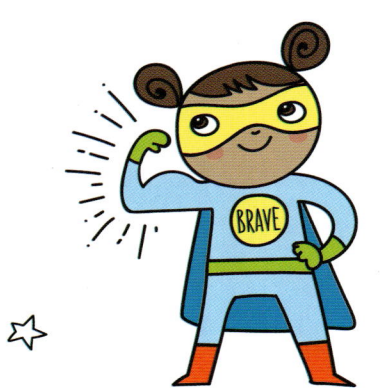

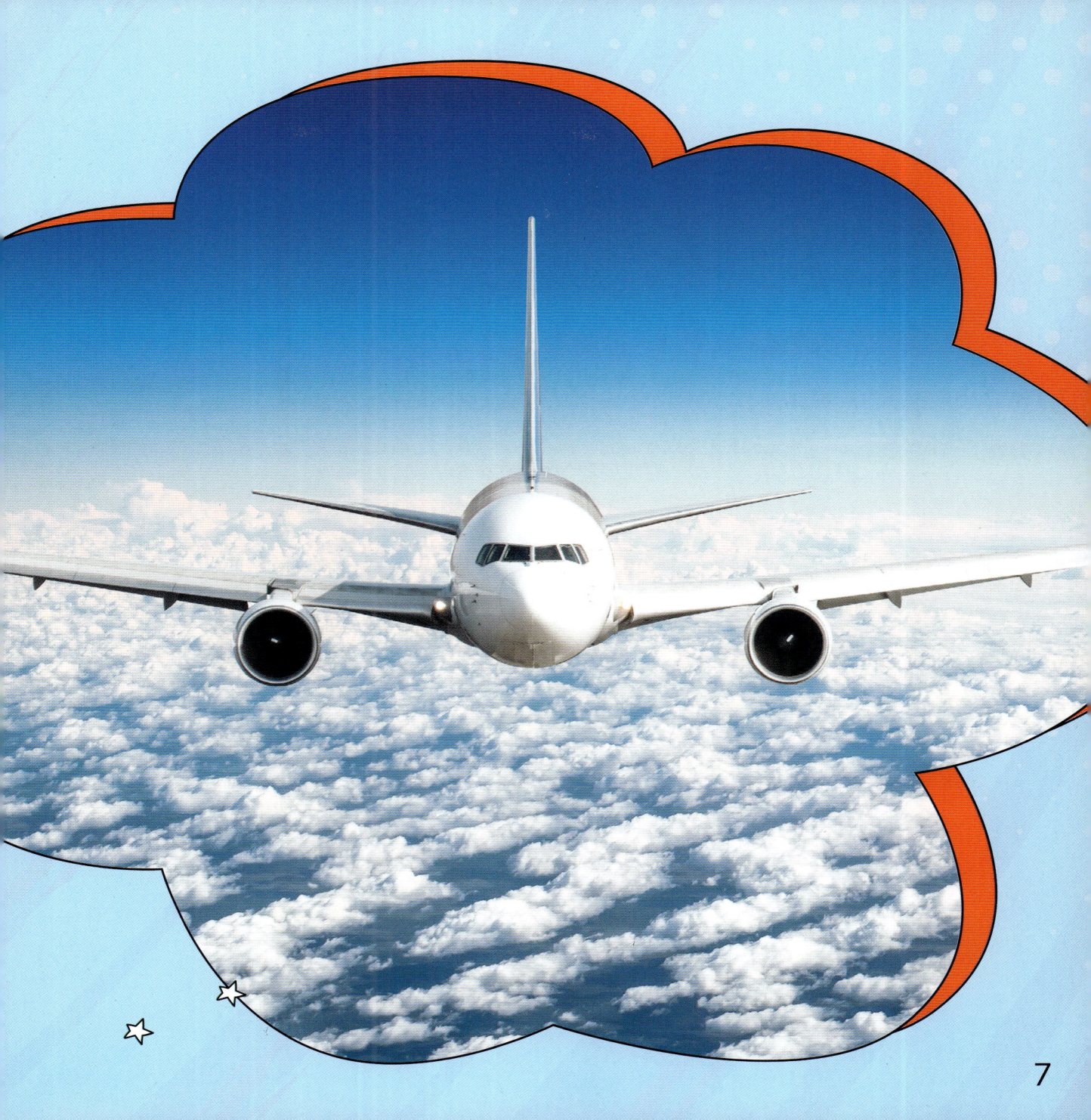

Many people work together to keep the plane safe. **Air traffic controllers** use equipment that shows them how many planes are in the sky. They also watch for changes in the weather. Controllers talk to the **pilot** during the flight.

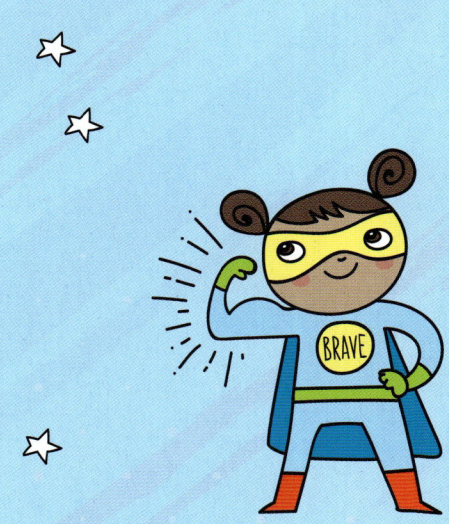

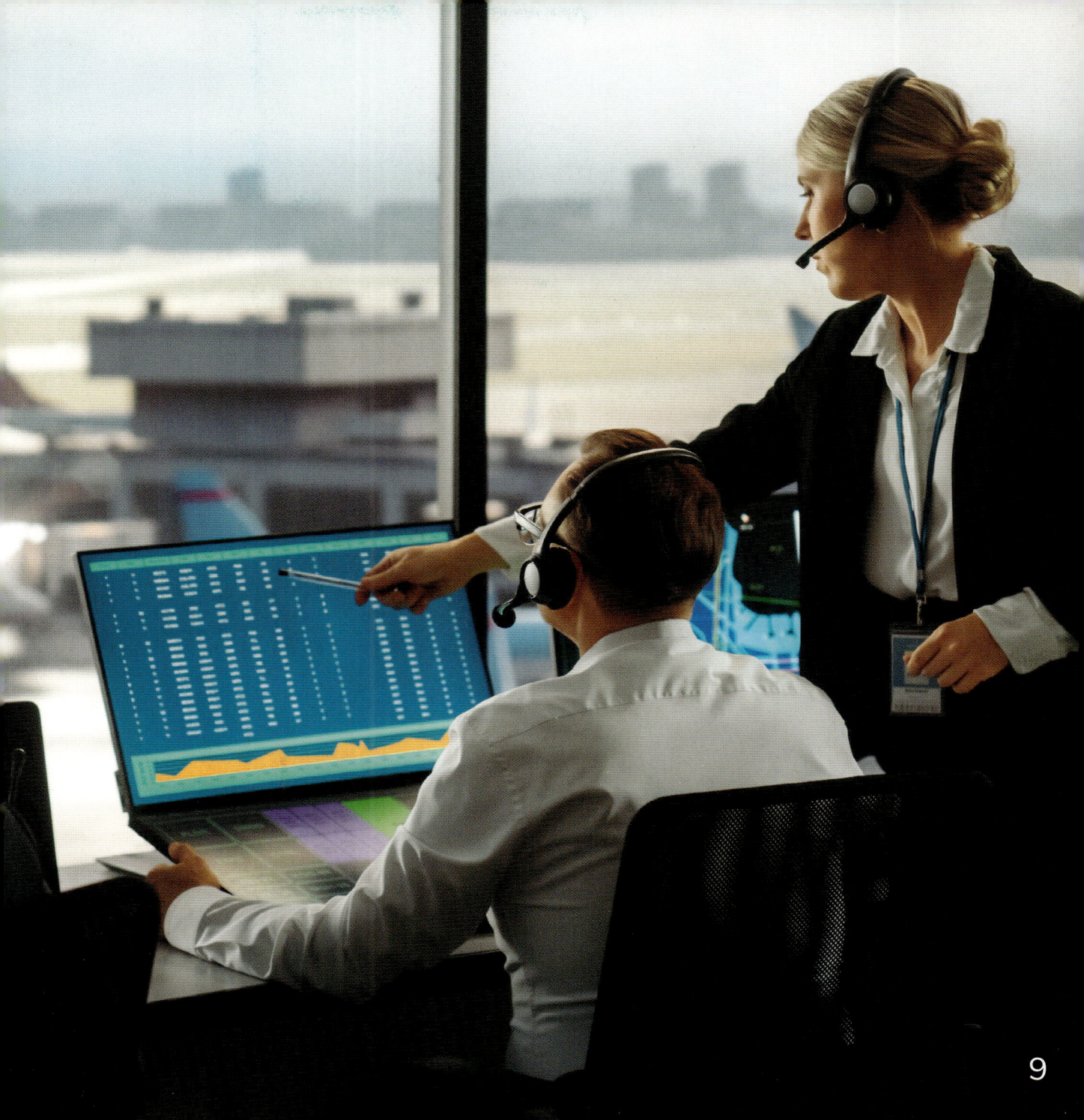

People on the plane keep it safe too. Pilots know all about the plane. They check it before take-off. They know how to use the plane's **instruments** and controls.

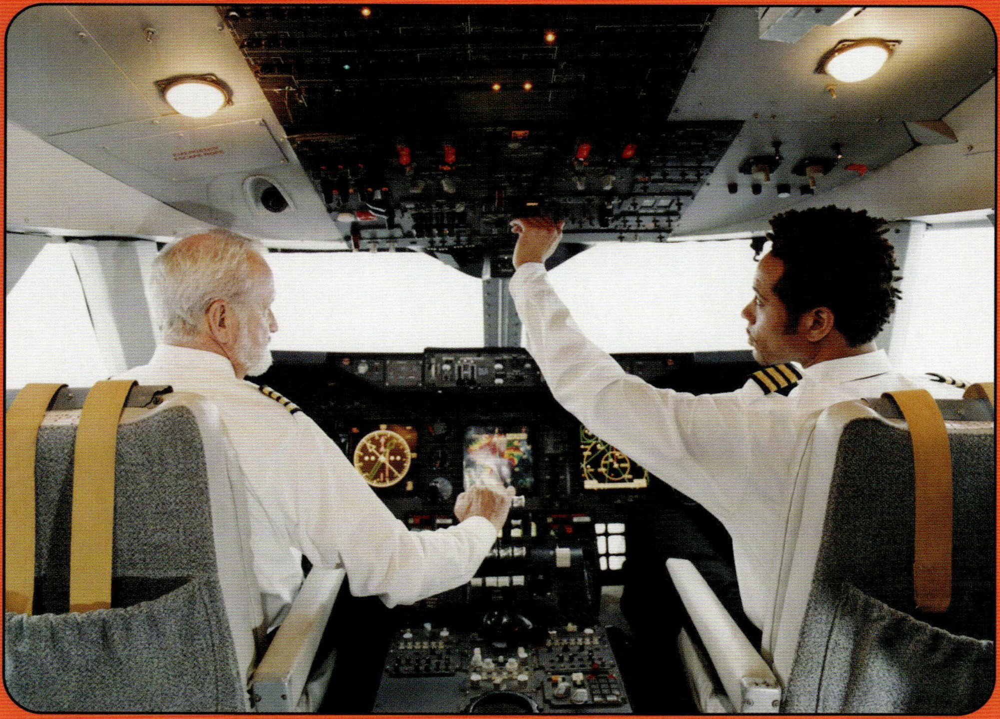

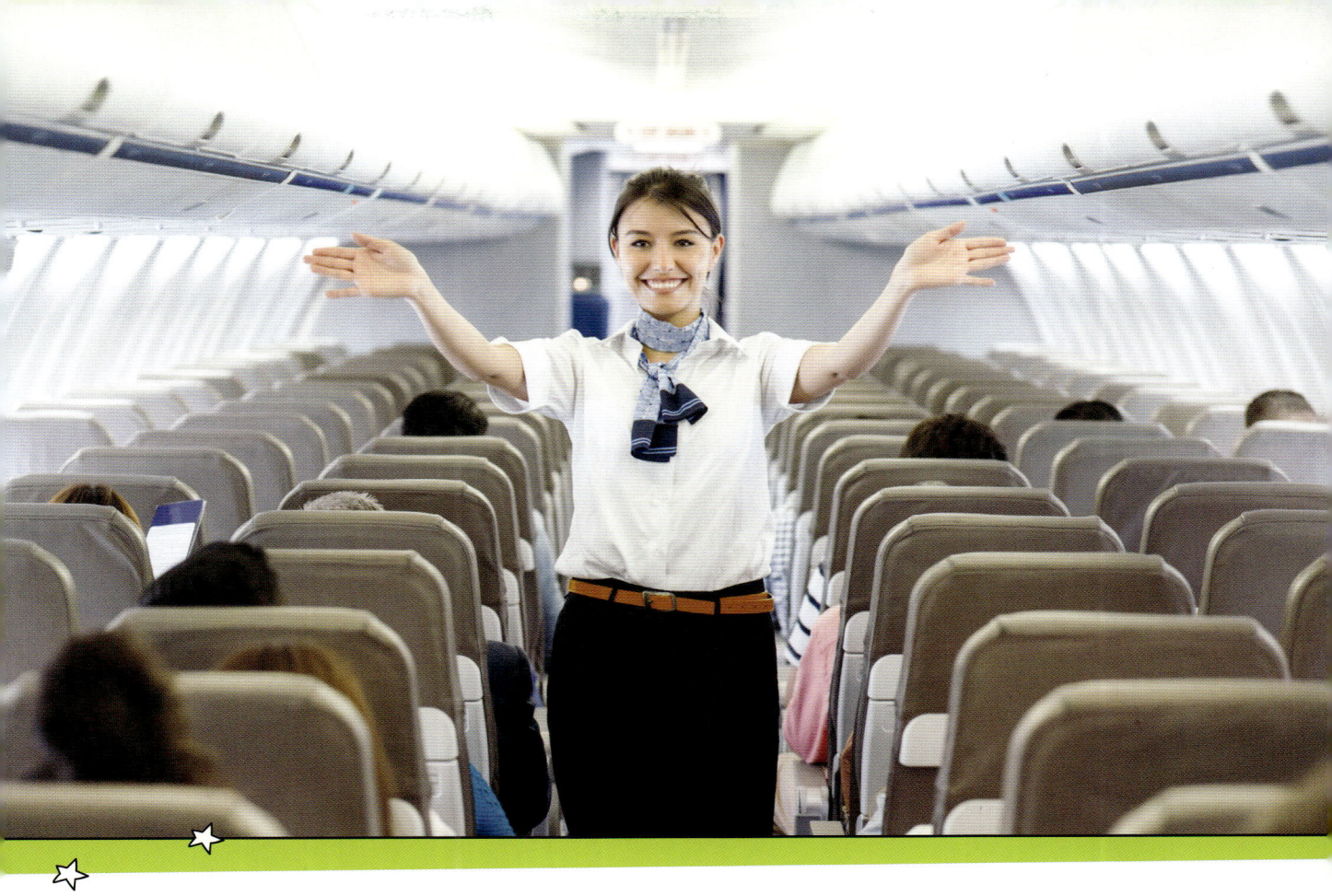

Flight attendants keep **passengers** comfortable and safe. They know what to do in an emergency. If you have questions, they can help. Ask away!

CALMING YOUR FEARS

Flying is more fun when you feel calm. Planning ahead helps. Pack a **carry-on bag**. Take an activity to keep busy. Add a favourite snack in case you get hungry.

You'll feel better if your body feels well too. It is normal for your ears to get blocked during a flight. If that happens, try chewing gum to help them clear up.

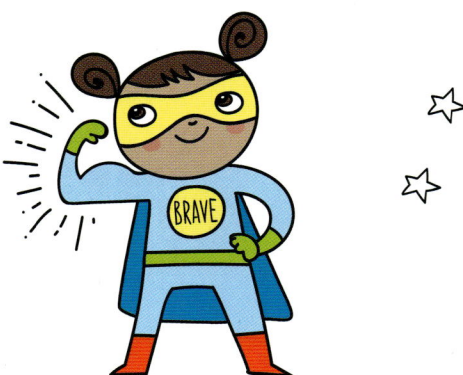

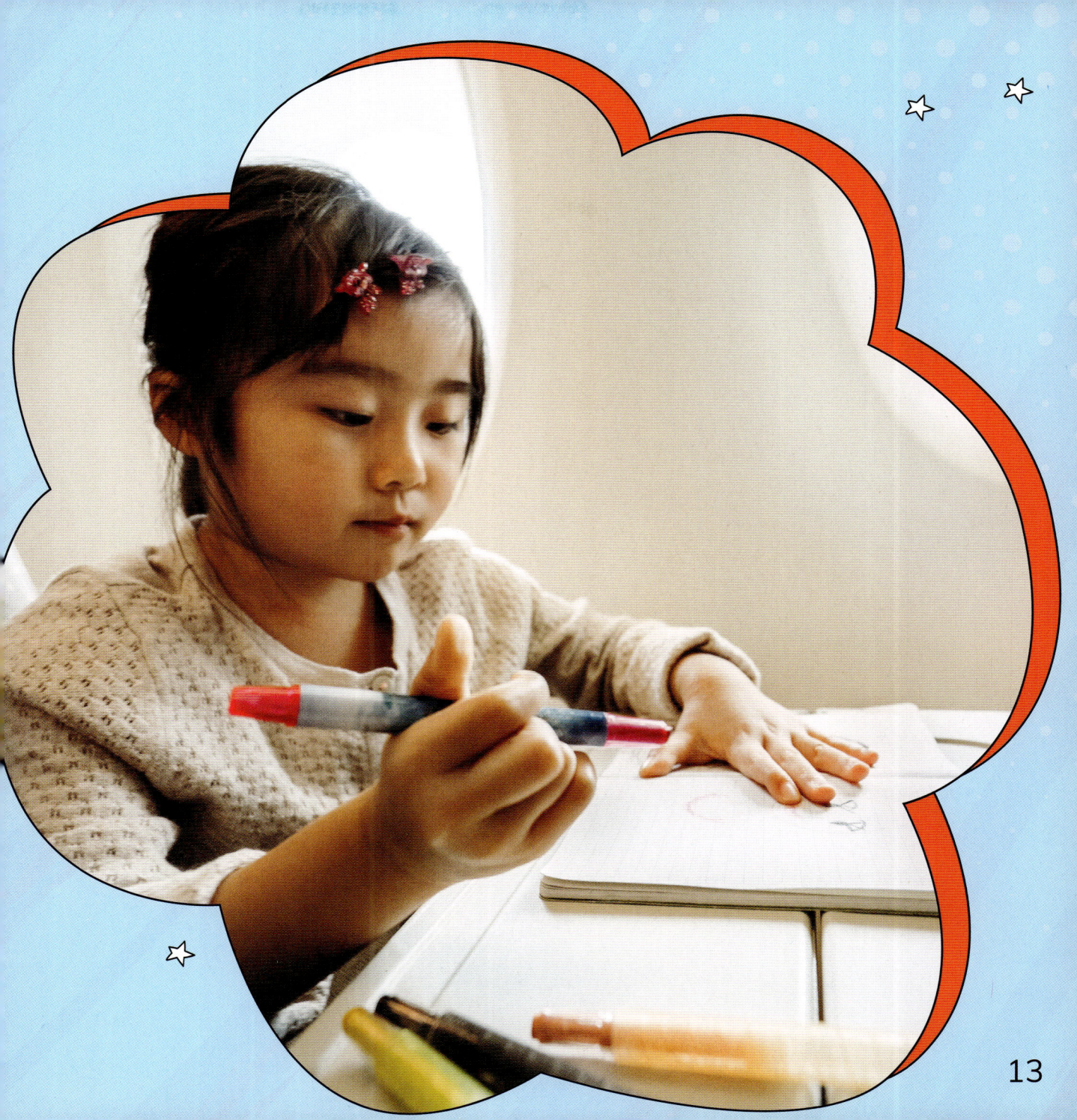

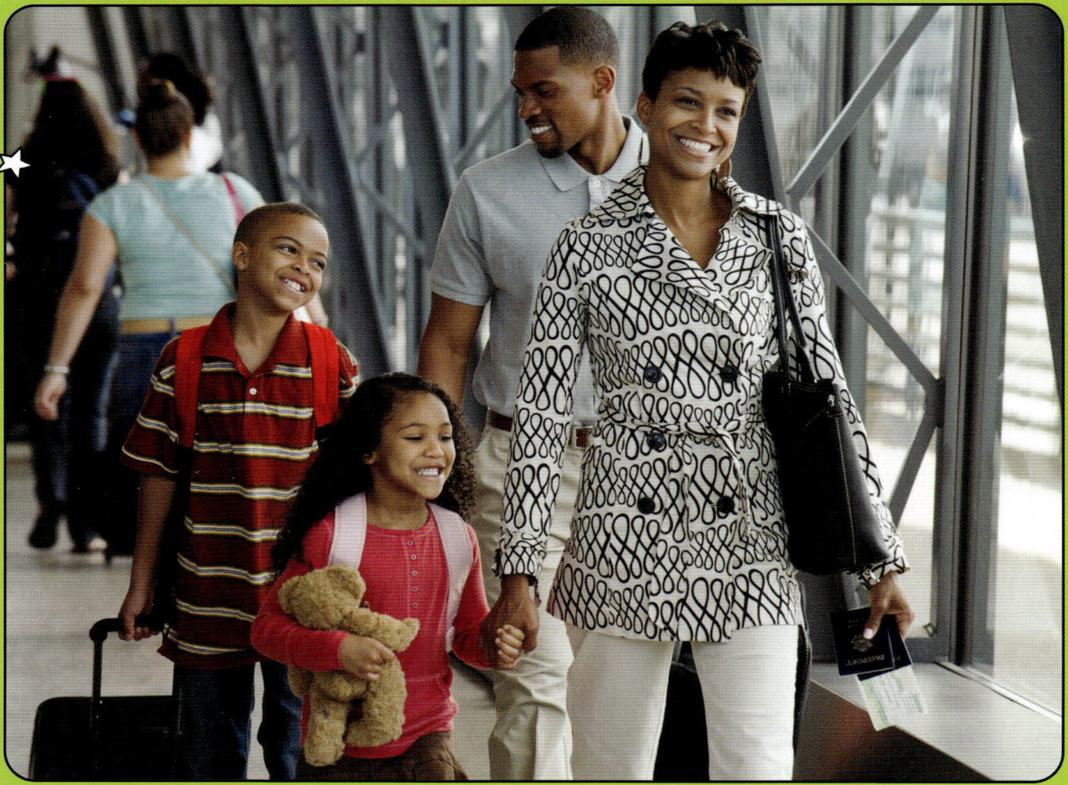

Are you someone who doesn't like waiting at the airport? If so, use your **imagination** to pass the time. Make up stories about where people are going.

Maybe you are more worried about being on the plane. You can use your imagination there too. Close your eyes. Pretend you are on a train or a bus.

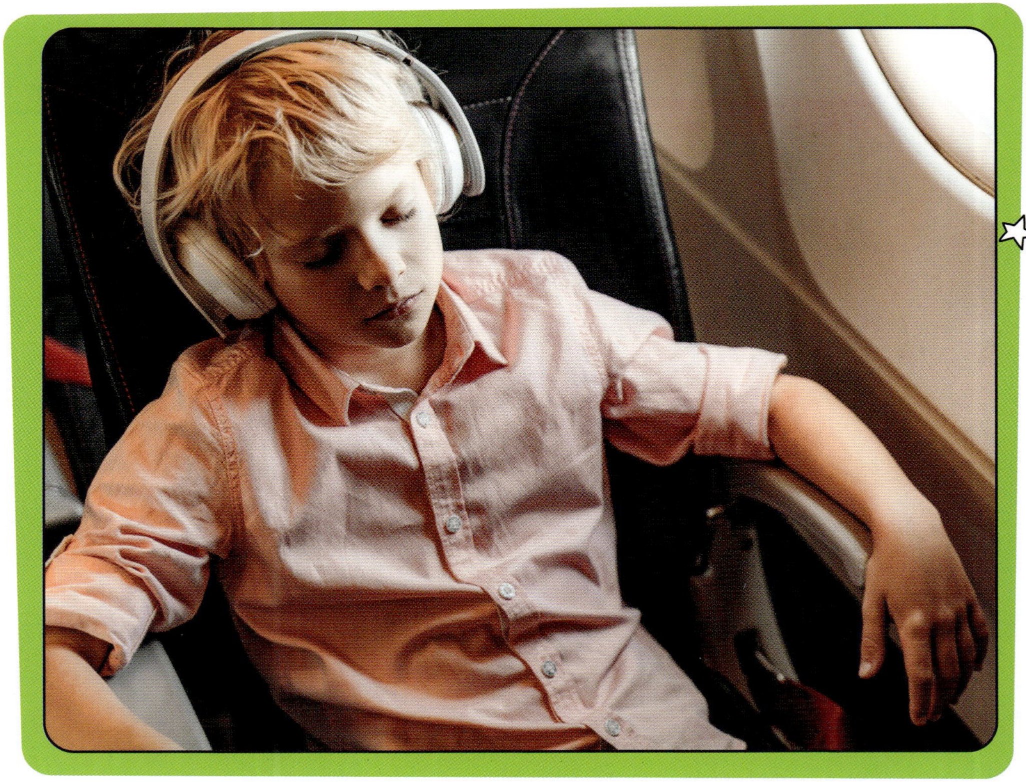

You might not get rid of all your fear. But there are plenty of other things to focus on during a flight. Look out the window at the clouds. Watch a film up in the air. Have a tasty in-flight snack. Staying busy will help you to stay calm.

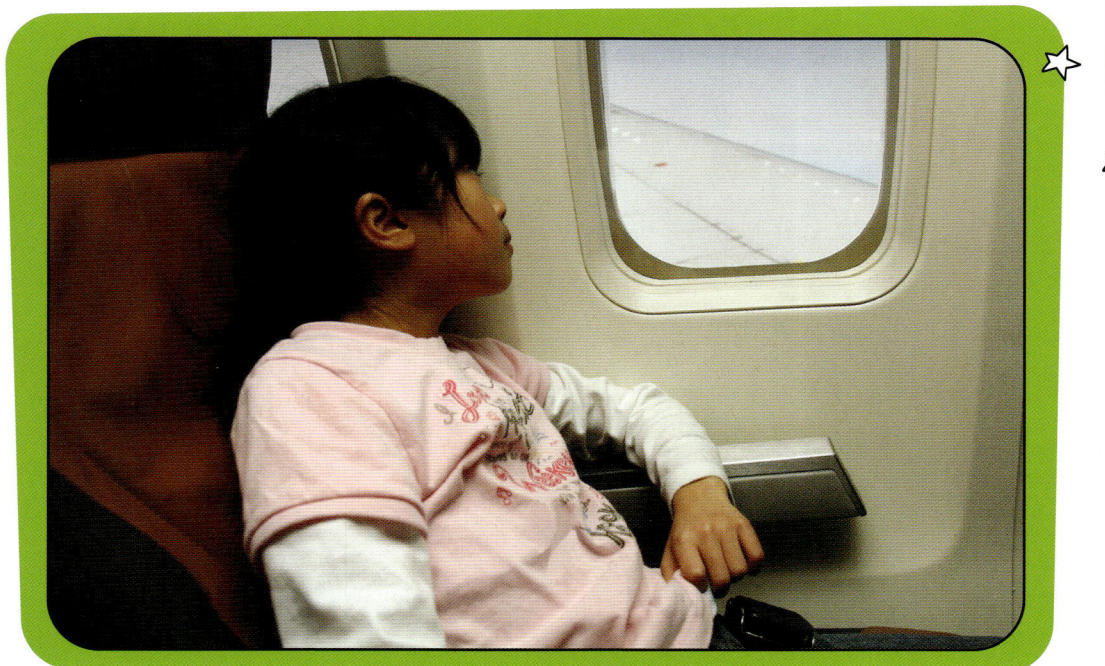

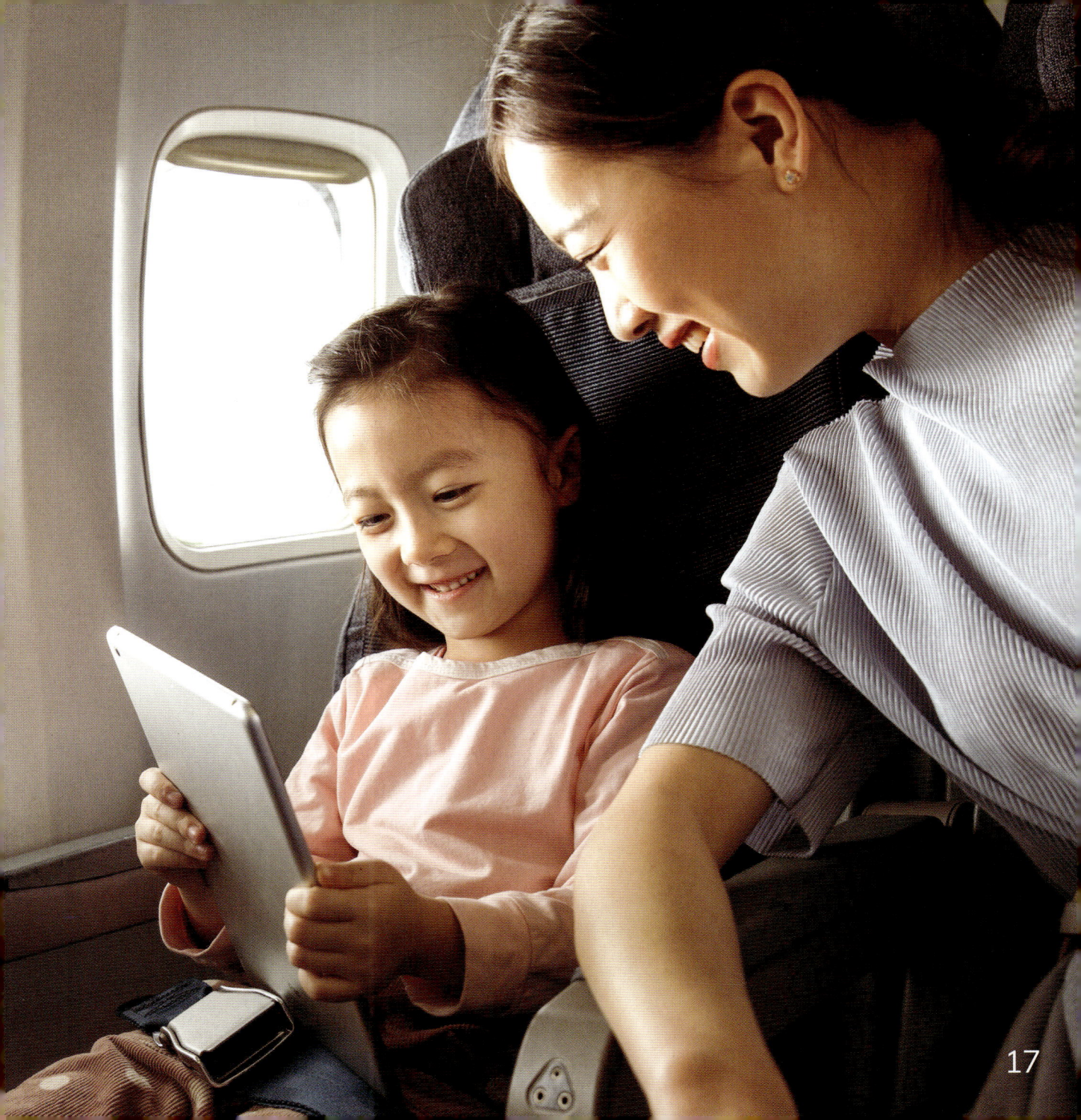

ENJOY THE RIDE

Are you still nervous about flying? That's only natural. Are you a bit excited? That's normal too.

With simple steps, you can stay calm. You can plan to enjoy the flight. And you can trust the people who work on planes. They care about keeping you safe.

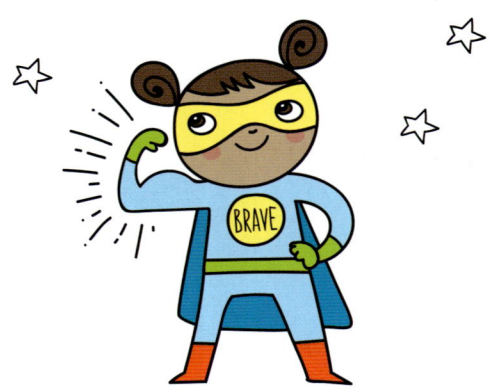

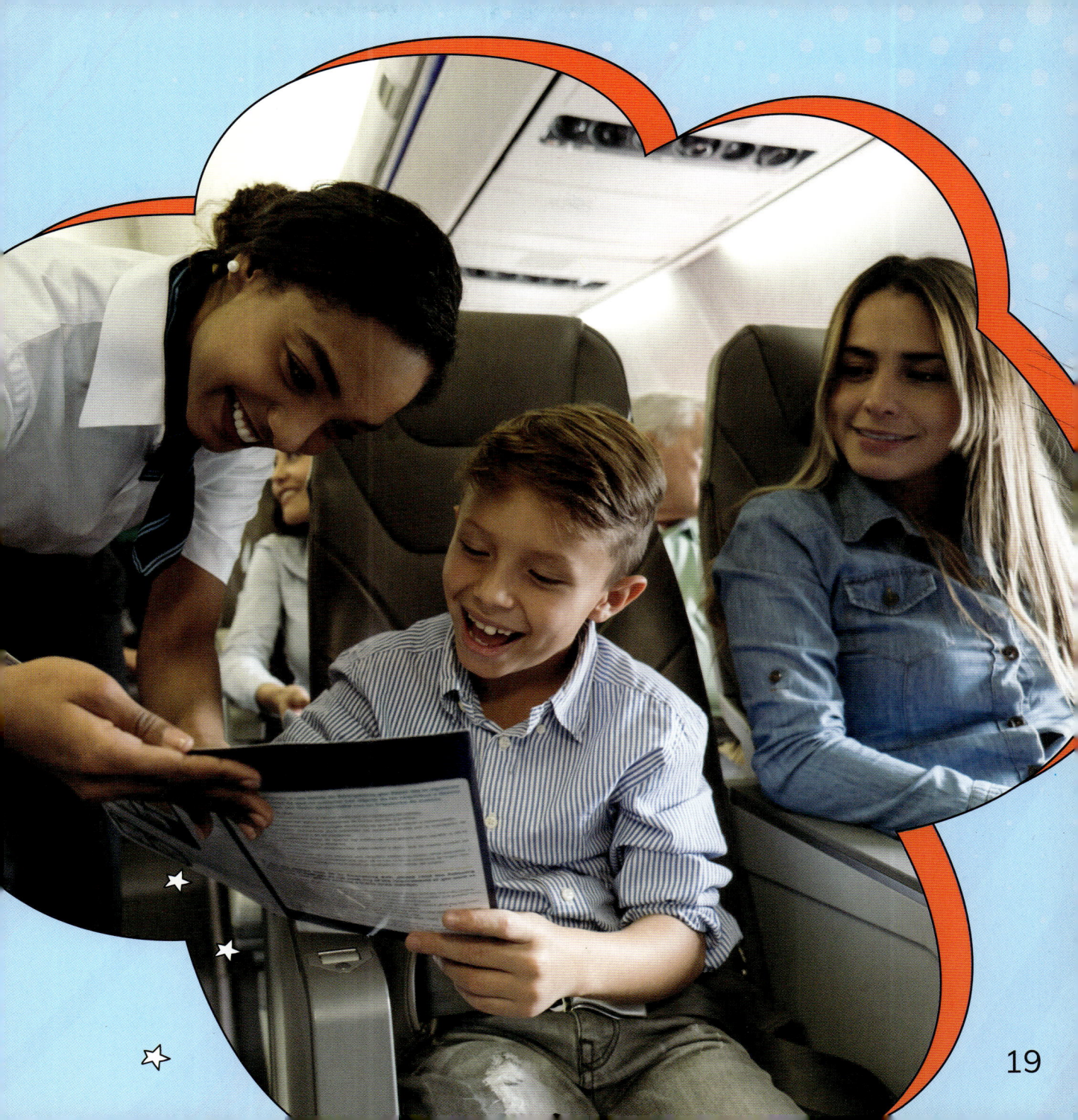

PACK A CARRY-ON BAG

Practise packing a carry-on bag for your flight. That way, you'll be ready for the real thing.

What you need

- small rucksack or other bag
- small toys and games
- books
- notebook
- pencil
- pre-packaged snacks

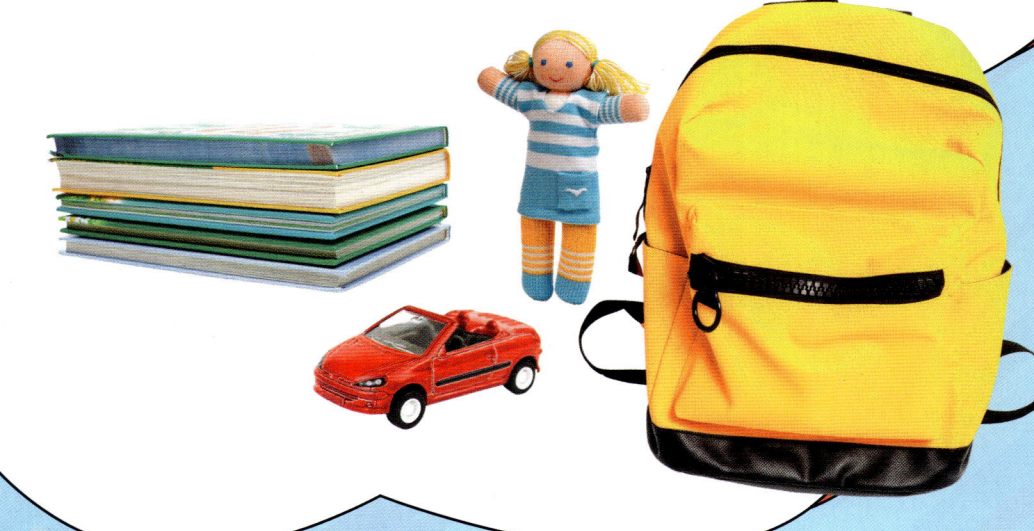

What to do

1. Find a small rucksack or other bag.

2. Gather a few toys and games that would be fun to have during the flight.

3. Gather one or two books, a notebook and a pencil.

4. Gather a few pre-packaged snacks, such as crackers and biscuits, that do not need to be kept in the fridge.

5. Look over your collected items. Decide which ones to take and which you could leave at home.

6. Pack the bag with the items you want to take.

7. Close the bag and try carrying it around. If your bag feels light, you could add a couple more items. If it feels too heavy, take a few things out.

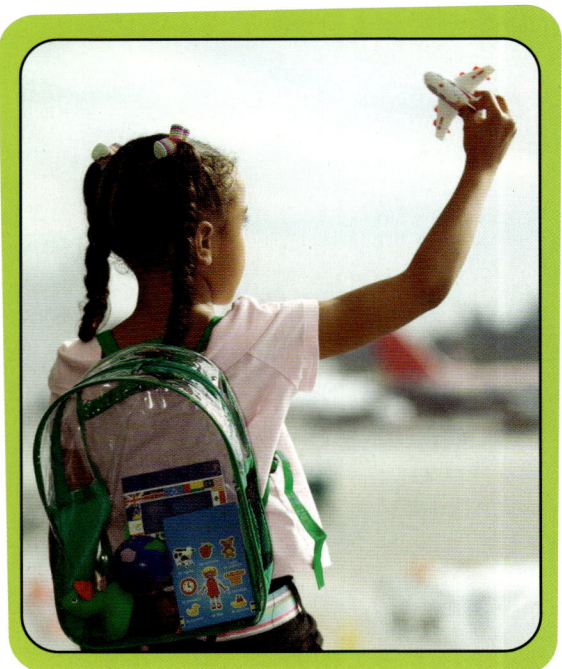

GLOSSARY

air traffic controller person who helps direct pilots from the ground

carry-on bag small piece of luggage that a passenger can carry onto an aeroplane

flight attendant person who helps passengers and serves food and drinks on an aeroplane

imagination ability to form pictures in your mind of things that are not present or real

instrument tool that gets information

passenger person who travels on an aeroplane, train or other vehicle

pilot person who flies a plane

take-off moment when an aeroplane leaves the ground and begins to fly

FIND OUT MORE

BOOKS

All About Worries and Fears, Felicity Brooks (Usborne, 2022)

How a Plane Works (Peep Inside), Lara Bryan (Usborne, 2020)

My Mixed Emotions: Learn to love your feelings, Elinor Greenwood (DK Children, 2018)

WEBSITES

www.bbc.co.uk/bitesize/topics/znhmwty/articles/z4q4bdm
Learn more about feelings and emotions.

www.bbc.co.uk/bitesize/topics/zvb76v4/articles/zk7qf4j
Learn more about what happens at the airport.

INDEX

activities 12, 14–16

air traffic controllers 8

chewing gum 12

engines 6

feelings 4, 12, 18

flight attendants 11

pilots 8, 10

snacks 12, 16

staying calm 12, 16, 18

wings 6

ABOUT THE AUTHOR

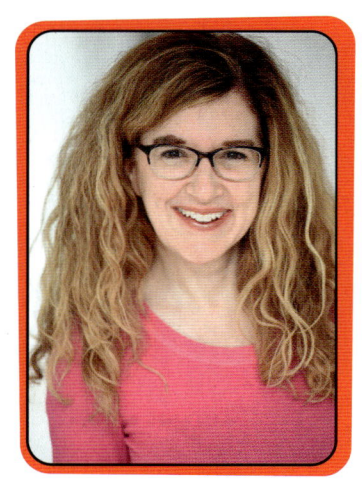

photo by Dan Doyle

Heather E. Schwartz has written hundreds of children's books. She gets nervous before flying, but loves looking out of the window when the plane is in the air. She lives in New York, USA, with her husband, two kids and two cats called Stampy and Squid.